CREATING
Healthy Life HABITS

Easy Tools for GETTING STARTED NOW

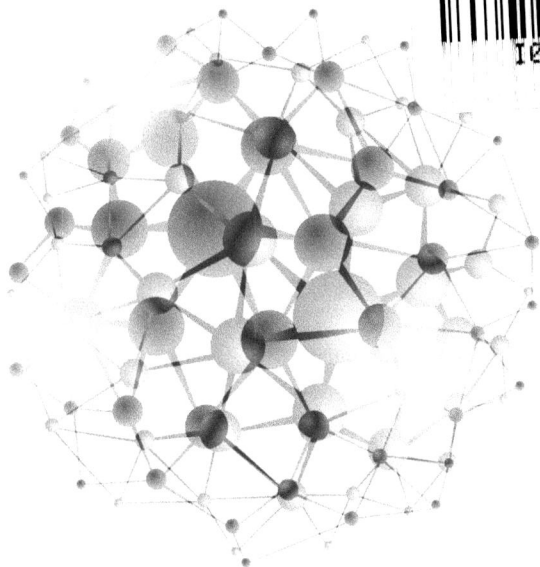

I0091480

Mandy Napier BSc (Hons)

Mandy Napier's
MINDSET
for Success®
EMPOWERMENT. ACTION. RESULTS.

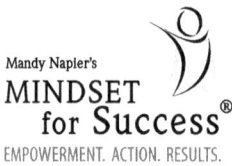

Graphic Design & Layout: Go-Enki.com.

Printed in Australia

First Printing, 2015

ISBN 978-0-9942316-0-4

Creating Healthy Life Habits: Your Guide to Getting Started Now / Mandy Napier BSc (Hons)

"I go back to this book time and time again to re motivate myself when I am stuck or to check out where I am stuck in life. It is easy to read and is full of insights and tools to help me on my journey.

"It reminds me that some habits I have developed are not working for me and they sneak back into my day now and then. I can change these habits with perseverance and awareness. This book gives me the tools to create change, stay motivated and to keep working on my life to get the best results for me. This means I am happier and my relationships improve because I am happier!

"I am a strong believer in mind over matter, being responsible for myself and my actions. If I set my mind on a positive path, being active with my health and wellbeing with tools I use from this book I am happier and more motivated with a mindset for my own personal success in life. Thank you for this valuable resource."

Sally Margan, Branxton, NSW

"One thing I've learned from Mandy Napier and from this book is how amazing setting goals can be. Having an idea, which turns into a picture and is virtually 'in my face' or stuck on my office door so that I can constantly be reminded of this goal that I'm going to achieve. Setting goals with a target, time frame and making them realistic makes them so much easier to achieve and gives me so much joy when the goals are fulfilled. I feel blessed every day in knowing the great results I am getting with your help and constant guidance."

Kellie Payne CFP, RetireInvest Proprietor

"As an optometrist I really identified with your use of 'vision' throughout the book. Vision, clarity and focus are words that really resonate with me and I am sure many others. Visualisation is the beginning point and the emerging science of Neuro-Plasticity gives us the 'OK' to make changes! My advice to someone picking up the book for the first time would be… Really take the time to read through the book. Don't rush it. Take time to stop and contemplate. Read it with a pen and paper...use the pen to make your actions real. This will make goal setting happen!"

Adrian Bell, Optometrist

"My admiration and respect for Mandy's professionalism and dedication to serving her clients' needs, without sacrificing her own, has only grown since we have reconnected in our current industry. She consistently invests in her own ongoing personal and professional development, striving to be her very best across all areas of her life and succeeding. Her clients benefit enormously from her continual growth and quest for even better resources and techniques. In addition to working with individuals, Mandy runs workshops, webinars and in-house training. She is also in demand as an inspiring guest speaker. The positive impact of Mandy's work is rippling out across the Sunshine Coast community and wider, as achieving success with each individual affects many. She has also contributed her time and expertise to the triathlete community, assisting with fine-tuning the mindset necessary for sporting success."

Sue Lester, Coach, Speaker, Author

"This book is something you cannot put down if you are into improving yourself or others around you. It looks at some great ways to drill down into who we really are and how to better our thinking. I love the Habit Changer Plan, which takes commitment, but works."

Darren Ide, Realway Property Consultants, Caloundra

"After reading the book I discovered that we can choose to be who or whatever we want to be. First, we have to be ready to accept change to see where we want to go and the person we want to be. It will take discipline and commitment - so does life! So why not live the life of your choosing?"

Colin Shurey, Premier1 Pest Control

"After reading Creating Healthy Life Habits so much of its content made me really think about my life and the habits I have developed over many years… some good and some not so good.

"What I liked about the book is that it gave me the direction that enabled me to start on the path to creating the habits that I wanted in my life.

"Even the most motivated people can find it hard to change their habits… Having been a highly motivated person myself for many years from competing at a high level in Ironman Triathlons, 100km running and completing 53 marathons, I have struggled over the last few years with changing my habits that I really wanted to change but did not have the insights to make it happen.

"I have had the pleasure of knowing Mandy both personally and professionally over the last 20 years. I have seen how Mandy has not only evolved herself, but has been able to channel her learnings with others who are struggling in their life… and that includes me.

"One of the key learnings I took from the book was the Watch Your Language! chapter. For a long time I was beating myself up constantly about who I used to be and what I used to achieve compared to who I am now and what I was achieving now. All I was really doing was poisoning my own mind and body. I am now more careful with my self-talk."

Mignon Auguszczak, PERICOACH Regional Account Manager, QLD/NT/New Zealand

"Mandy has written some sage advice in this powerful little book. I have seen Mandy in recent times and she does what she teaches. A lot of topics are covered. The highest human good is peace of mind and that comes when we are happy. Treasure your mind as a gift so please look after it. Understand 'how we do one thing in life is how we do everything'. This statement resonated with me and I realised that we are usually the biggest obstacle to our success. It all starts with a decision to change something that isn't working. Mandy can help you to get your mindset the way it will help you best. She has a number of techniques that will make your life more effective. The pain of discipline is a lot lighter than the pain of regret."

Steve Power, Power Financials

"For someone lucky enough to have natural survival and tenacity it is even harder to reach out and ask for help – thank you so much Mandy for guiding me to dig a little deeper and find the confidence and wisdom to be better than just 'getting by'."

Jen Hope

TABLE OF CONTENTS

INTRODUCTION

*'We first make our habits and
then our habits make us.'*
~ John Dryden

*'Who am I?' 'I am your constant companion. I am
your greatest help or heaviest burden. I will push you
onwards or drag you down to failure. I am completely
at your command. Half the things you do you might
just as well turn over to me and I will do them quickly
and correctly. I am easily managed; you must merely
be firm with me. Show me exactly how you want
something done and after a few lessons I will do it
automatically. I am the servant of all great men and
women and, alas, of all failures as well. Those who are
great, I have made great. Those who are failures, I have
made failures. I am not a machine, though I work with
the precision and repetition of a machine, plus the
intelligence of a human. You may run me for profit or
run me for ruin, it makes no difference to me. Take me,*

train me, be firm with me, and I will place the world at your feet. Be easy with me and I will destroy you. Who am I? I am a Habit.'

Anonymous Riddle

Habit: (Definition)

'A settled or regular tendency or practice, especially one that is hard to give up.'

My guess is, if you're reading this, you are probably experiencing some challenges making changes in your life. Humans are creatures of habit, which is one reason why you may be struggling! Nevertheless, I bet you know someone who has effortlessly given up smoking or embarked on a healthy eating regime. You may even know them intimately! But why is it that some people find change harder than others?

There's not just one answer. Yet my intention is that when you read this book, you will uncover crucial keys that will help you seamlessly make the changes you desire. The intention of this book is to:

› Help you gain a deeper understanding of yourself and your mind, so that you can make more conscious choices, create healthy habits and the changes you desire in your life.

› Give you useful tools, ideas and strategies to help you release unwanted habits and create new and desirable ones.

WHY IS IT HARD TO CHANGE?

Humans are an intriguing species, capable of amazing feats; yet too often we never fully achieve our goals and dreams. On the one hand we can land men on the moon, build space stations and send satellites around the world, yet in lesser tasks such as pursuing our individual health and weight loss goals, we often fail miserably!

DID YOU KNOW?

Most New Year's Resolutions fail. In a 2013 Forbes report research from the University of Scranton, they concluded that only 8% of people achieve their New Year's goals. That means a whopping 92% fail!

Most diets fail. Have you ever been on one, lost weight and then put it back on? Many statistics state that around 90% of all diets fail with people often regaining more weight than before they dieted.

A large percentage of Australians are overweight and diabetes is on the increase. Why is this so? Could this be more evidence proving what we know: that most people struggle with creating healthy habits and sticking with them, never achieving the level of health that they desire?

DO YOU HAVE POOR HABITS YOU WOULD LIKE TO CHANGE?

> - If so, what do you specifically want to change? Imagine the benefits.

> - Have you tried to change and fallen back into your old habits?

> - Are you feeling stuck and frustrated, failing yet again?

> - What major goals have you started in your life and then given up? Is it your health, a business venture or an exercise routine? What do you think went wrong?

> - Are you eager to live the extraordinary life you deserve, but can't quite do what's necessary to make it happen?

THEN, THIS BOOK IS ABSOLUTELY FOR YOU!

The tools and techniques that I share in this book are the ones I have used in my life to make significant changes. They are those I teach my clients, to their great success. When you use these tools consistently, they will help you 'get out of your own way'. You will be empowered to create new habits, implement new strategies and with continual focus and action, will see your results change. When you invest in yourself, you are investing in your future. When you understand yourself and open up to a world of limitless possibilities, you will take charge of your life, your destiny and step forward purposefully into the direction of your dreams.

Life is not a rehearsal for something else. It is the real thing.

Creating new, healthy habits, as denoted in the opening quote, is a fundamental key to your future success and happiness. In the words of Stephan Widmer, a friend of mine and a highly successful international swim coach: *'Motivation is what gets you started. Habit is what keeps you going.'*

The creation of healthy habits lies at the cornerstone of all achievements and successes in life. Good habits help you create all the other key ingredients necessary for making change: clarity, self-belief, consistent action, focus, courage and commitment.

ACTION STEP:

Make a list of your good habits and your not-so-good habits. Now write down what behaviours and actions you would like to replace these 'not so good habits' with.

Would you like to get up earlier and exercise, rather than sleeping in? Would you like to eat fresher, healthy fruit and vegetables instead of turning to unhealthier, yet convenient fast foods?

Your next action now is to compose a few sentences about how your life will be once you have made these changes and created your new habits.

Did you do that or just read it?

This step is important in creating your change, so stop right now and make sure you have completed the above action step!

WHY DO WE FIND IT HARD TO CHANGE?

As humans, we are hardwired to keep ourselves safe. When we were hunter-gatherers, the world was a foreboding place.

Our focus was on survival, finding food and keeping out of harm's way.

Today, our lives are full of modern conveniences, books and Google to help us in every aspect of our lives. Yet we still struggle to make positive changes and to find that elusive 'happiness', perhaps the ultimate currency in life.

Whenever we embark on something new, like changing a habit or starting a healthy eating regime, we have to navigate around our inner gatekeeper, whose mission it is to protect us from harm. To assist us in survival when our 'flight or fight' mechanism kicks in, stress chemicals – adrenalin and cortisol – are released to help us encounter the possible danger. The physical reaction that occurs causes us to 'feel' something, usually fear or doubt. In some people, this causes a knot or butterflies in the stomach, a sick feeling, sweaty palms or a racing heart.

Most people let these feelings stop them in their tracks, interpreting them to mean they can't do something. They may feel the fear or doubt and hear a voice that says 'it's too difficult', 'perhaps this isn't for me'… or 'I can't do this.'

To make matters worse, awful memories arise from some of our past experiences that cloud the present moment and set the scene for our future. Negative thoughts attract more negative thoughts, which shape our future. Not the best recipe for success! Consequently, all dreams go by the wayside and goals are abandoned as we let our past experiences extinguish new possibilities.

WHAT HAPPENS WHEN YOU HIT AN OBSTACLE?

> What do you say to yourself?

> Do you use the obstacle as evidence or an excuse to prove a deep-held, often false belief? Perhaps hearing that inner critic saying, 'I can't do this,' or 'I'm not good enough'?

> Do you normally view obstacles as being 'in the way' or being 'on the way'?

> Do you find a way around the obstacle or do you give up?

> Do you see obstacles as opportunities to learn and grow?

The disturbing truth is, unless you are someone with firmly built programs called 'discipline' and 'persistence' and your internal dial is set towards success, you will get stuck and at times stall. Unless you do something to resolve the underlying blocks, your 'issues', you may be one of the 92% who never achieve their New Year's resolutions and goals.

If you didn't have an amazing upbringing filled with inspiring people, positive encouragement, fuelled by beliefs in an abundant universe... with a strong feeling that you can be, do and have anything, well, you will have some limiting beliefs and old patterns to clear out. The good news is that the tools herein, once implemented and continually used, will make it easier.

> *Our past can trap us, holding us*
> *like a prisoner in our life.*

Susan (name changed for confidentiality) came to see me because she was battling with her weight and was sick and tired of her roller coaster ride of yo-yo dieting. Every time she lost a few kilos, she put them back on. (Plus some!) She had tried every new diet available. Having failed miserably on numerous occasions, she knew she needed to do something radically different and find a permanent solution to this problem.

*She made a decision, called **Mindset for Success** and booked her first appointment.*

During our work together, we uncovered limiting beliefs she wasn't aware of. When she was young she recalled being told repeatedly by her well-meaning mother, 'you must finish the food on your plate'. (Can you relate to this?) Consequently, whether or not she was really hungry, she always ate everything on her plate. This belief was ingrained into her subconscious mind. Every time she ate and cleared her plate, she added fuel to this belief, which then became a habit she felt powerless to break.

We also discovered a deep-seated belief around a fear of being successful, and more specifically, a fear of becoming slim and attractive.

After our process work and with some effective new tools and strategies to try out, she soon recognised and released her limiting beliefs. I taught her new healthier eating strategies. As she noticed the results, she became more empowered to continue. Slowly, her life started to change in positive ways. Not only did she start to create healthier habits around food and eating, so she lost weight, her self-esteem and confidence also rose, allowing her to transform many other areas of her life.

The best news is, if Susan can change, you can too. But you must want to change. If necessary, seek a consultation with a professional to help you make the changes you desire.

Another reason people find it hard to change is that we are creatures of habit. We are hardwired to be kept safe and tend to fall back into the easiest, most comfortable way of doing things. It is so much easier to take the easy path, the one we have travelled down many times before.

Is it easier to sleep in on a dark, cold morning, or to leap out of bed and go to the gym when you hate exercising? What happens when you are tired after a long day at work? Do you tend to grab a take-away, or prepare a healthy meal?

Making changes and doing new things in life, takes effort, persistence, will and focus to succeed. It's hard work. Naturally, most people prefer the easy way, the familiar and the comfortable.

When you repeatedly do the same thing frequently, you literally create a well-worn path. There is a phrase in Neuro-Science, 'what fires together, wires together'.

Your bodily functions, attitudes and learned skills are all keyed into your subconscious mind and stored as programs. Habits become woven into your brain and define what you do.

This is a key point in understanding why you may have found it difficult to make changes and to maintain them. The secret to changing a habit is to change it! To challenge yourself to do things differently and better; take small steps and persist. Unfortunately, this often feels like hard work to many people!

Our minds are geared to move towards pleasure and away from pain.

It has been proven by social researchers that our minds are geared to make choices to move towards pleasure and away from pain. We tend to prefer instant gratification over long term gain. Would you like to receive your wage at the end of the week or at the end of the year with a ten per cent bonus?

We often say we don't feel like doing something. It doesn't feel pleasurable at that moment in time, so we never get going. Can you recall a time when you intended to do something positive and talked yourself out of it?

HAVE YOU EVER BEEN GUILTY OF:

> Hitting the snooze button on the alarm and sleeping in, because you didn't really feel like getting up on a cold morning and going to the gym? Telling yourself you will start tomorrow?

> Settling down on the sofa for a few minutes and watching TV instead all night, instead of studying or reading an educational book?

> Watching a good movie surrounded by comfort food or a beer instead of choosing a healthy herbal tea?

> Grabbing a take-away because you tell yourself you are too tired to prepare a healthy meal and you will start your healthy eating plan tomorrow?

Can you see how you have been caught in this pattern and given in to a choice that is more pleasurable at that moment in time? Choosing instant gratification over long-term gain?

Humans tend to lose focus frequently.

I have heard it said many times that the typical person loses focus every 6-10 seconds. So, if you don't continually decide to refocus frequently, you will lose your focus, yet keeping focus often requires hard work! And honestly, who really likes continual hard work?

According to the National Science Foundation, we have around 50,000 thoughts a day.

Ninety-five per cent of these thoughts are repeated daily and are a reflection of the beliefs and attitudes that we hold.

Most people have no idea of the internal chatter going on inside their heads, or have any idea that they can take charge of the chatter.

There are very few classes that help you understand how your mind works.

A key to taking charge of your life is to become aware of what you are doing, understand how you think, feel and act… discover what triggers your behaviour… then you can start to change your actions, behaviours and results.

By integrating my tools and systems in this book into your actions and thoughts, you will start to take charge of your life.

Have you ever stopped to write down your thoughts? To spend time observing what you say to yourself? Have you questioned your behaviour, considering carefully before behaving in a certain way?

Do you know what emotions you feel, or where in your body you feel them? How many emotions could you even name?

Your thoughts and feelings govern your actions and behaviour, which in turn lead to your current results. When you understand yourself, when you have the right mind tools and use them, you will create your own winning formula… a mindset for success.

A MINDSET FOR SUCCESS MEANS:

> › You can dismantle the 'mental monsters' you have created in your head.

> › You can change those rambling negative thoughts that become habits of thought to better results.

> › You can use your conscious mind as a tool to tame the vast jungle of your subconscious mind.

> › You can take charge of your life and steer your ship towards the destination of your choice!

> › You will be equipped to ride smoothly over the bumps along the way.

> › Sometimes, an event, or experience in life is the catalyst for change.

MY STORY

As I reflect back on my life, certain catalysts and events stand out. Certain 'turning point' experiences, both bitter and sweet, mark the journey like beacons. Catalysts fuelled the choices I made and made me strong and determined.

I was born in England and at the age of 17 years, I left home to commence a University degree. Needing to supplement my studies as well as save for overseas travel, I found part-time work in the student union bar. Although student life on the whole was fun, there were tough times. Enduring the hardships of living frugally, being cold, tired and juggling late nights (whether studying or working), was all part of being a student I believed. However, it took great effort, determination, dedication, discipline and resilience to succeed.

Indeed, it would have been easier to give up when the going got tough; to not show up for work when I was exhausted and had assignments to finish; pulling out of my six month placement which was a complete nightmare, which at that time, seemed a questionable experience. But I didn't give up. I persisted because giving up wouldn't have been true to my aspirations.

After completing my four-year degree and a brief intense period of earning full-time money, I set off travelling. I eventually landed in Australia with a working visa. Experiencing sheep farms, picking tomatoes, grapes, peaches, oranges and even pumpkins and tomatoes, I immersed myself in the experiences. After more travelling and a four-year stint working in London, I eventually returned to Australia, married and became an

Australian citizen. This process was fast tracked so I could represent Australia in a triathlon, the culmination of a childhood dream.

At around the same time, I realised the sad reality that our relationship – once so beautiful – had developed into a very unhappy marriage. Suppressing this anguish and my deepest fears, I focussed on my career and sporting goal of representing Australia. After completing the first world's long course triathlon championships in Nice, France, then racing in Muncie, Illinois, the next stop for me was the Australian Ironman, held in Forster, NSW, where I succeeded in qualifying to compete at the World Championships: the gruelling Hawaiian Ironman race. This experience should have been the pinnacle of my sporting career, despite having an injury and developing a severe cough. Little did I know what this experience would have in store and what road it would eventually take me down.

It was not long after the Hawaiian Ironman that things started to get drastically worse. My marriage was in an irresolvable state, so I finally did what my intuition had been telling me to do for a long time. I left my husband, took a few possessions and moved out of our house. I was left in debt, with no house and no family in Australia. I was emotionally bruised, yet I felt that a dark cloud was released from around me, giving me a sense of freedom.

As I continued to do what I loved, training for more triathlons, I noticed strange things happening when I ran. Muscles pulled in opposite directions, which resulted in difficulty moving forward and left me in physical pain. I had no idea what was going on… and it was getting worse. One day I was running and the next, after a visit to a physiotherapist, I had to stop completely. This mysterious sport-stopping ailment took away the one thing I loved.

'Where to from here?' I asked myself. The first step was to find a health professional to fix my body and mind. This turned out to be an interesting and costly journey. Being unable to find a satisfactory mainstream solution to my health, I took an alternative path to healing, venturing down the road of personal development courses, healing modalities and transformational courses. I embraced the opportunity to learn more about myself and about personal development. New insights and knowledge helped me heal and became the catalyst that shaped my current life.

The more courses I did, the more insights I gained. More than this, I was startled with my findings. I realised that it's how we deal with our experiences that are crucial to our results, not the actual experience itself. It's the choices we make at critical times and how we view obstacles, setbacks and challenges that determine what we do next. It is at these times of crisis, or 'choice' points, that we either grow or shrink.

WHY IS IT HARD TO CHANGE

Believing that, as individuals, we are responsible for our circumstances, I knew deep down that I had somehow created my current poor state of health. I had no idea how, yet I knew that if I persisted and found the gold nuggets behind my experiences, I would discover the key to heal myself.

After much soul searching, many discussions and months of doing a plethora of weird and wonderful courses, I started to heal. My body became less knotted and I started participating in sport again. The most amazing thing was that I transformed other areas of my life that I wasn't even focussing on. What a great bonus!

During this time I uncovered patterns and programs that were lying like silent saboteurs waiting to block the door to success. I found limiting beliefs that I had unknowingly learnt when I was young. As I explored my dark corners and applied the tools and techniques I was taught, I revealed these long-held patterns and gradually transformed them. Just like upgrading the software in your computer, your results then change. And so I began to feel different, more energetic. I started to notice the world around me with new eyes. As I stepped into a new me, I felt revitalised; metaphorically reinventing myself in specific parts of my life. I began to shine again.

Even better, I knew that these proven tools were the key for transforming lives. If I could transform my health, find my ideal partner, change careers and create my own business, then these tools could help others make similar changes. I discovered an inner calm and clarity to my life. So it became my mission to help others change their past patterns, create new programs, healthy habits and transformations.

I now live a blessed life. I have an endearing husband. I live near the ocean – the place I dreamt of living near since I was a young girl in England. Saying goodbye to a successful career in travel, I opened the next chapter in life, establishing my business 'Mindset for Success'.

I now coach individuals to shine, teaching them transformational tools and powerful strategies for success. I help them become the best version of themselves, boosting their health, wellbeing and fulfilment, helping them find the ultimate currency in life, that of 'happiness'. Some of the tools are freely available on my website.

Subscribe today to receive monthly mindset tips and download a complimentary copy of 'Your Hidden Mind' at **www.mindsetforsuccess.com.au.**

ENERGY, SCIENCE AND YOU

THE UNSEEN WORLD

Now, for the best news… change is possible. If I can change and others can, you can too. You have unlimited potential! But don't just take my word for it, read the evidence backed by science. One of the greatest discoveries of this century, in my view, is that of **NEURO-PLASTICITY.** This means: the capacity of the brain to change itself, to recreate new pathways that create change.

It doesn't matter if you are broke, overweight, sick, or regularly sad. It doesn't matter if you are still looking for love, or if you have a dead end job. You can change. You have the potential to do whatever you desire and become the person you want to be.

Despite whatever the past has dealt you, it is 100% possible to change yourself, redesign your future and create something better for yourself.

Now this is going to sound a little weird, but bear with me. In the world of Quantum Physics, the findings of which has thrown traditional science upside down, all living things are fundamentally energy. Specifically, we are waves and particles of energy. Everything and everyone is connected, which means the world is a vast web of interconnected relationships.

If you are curious to read about Neuro-Plasticity and how your brain can adapt to new conditions and rewire itself, pick up a copy of *The Brain that Changes Itself* by Norman Doidge and *The Biology of Beliefs* by Dr Bruce Lipton.

Dr Lipton is a Cell Biology Professor who has given us profound insights into the fundamental interconnectedness of science and spirit. Your genes no longer have to be your destiny!

Research has now proven that thoughts, beliefs, emotions and attitudes profoundly influence the function of our cells, organs and immune system, processes that are vital to our health and overall sense of wellbeing.

Lipton's findings, as well as that of Dr Candace Pert (a neuroscientist), conclude that our DNA is controlled by signals from the environment (that is, everything outside the cell). This includes our positive and negative beliefs, our emotions and thoughts, which all have an impact upon cell membrane receptors.

Our thoughts and emotions can influence genetic expression of health or disease.

IS MATTER REAL?

The work of Masaru Emoto beautifully illustrates how the power of the mind can profoundly influence the appearance of observed crystalline formations in water molecules. From his book, *The Message from Water* he provides factual evidence that human vibrational energy, thoughts, words, ideas and music affect the molecular structure of water. This is the same water that comprises over 70% of a mature human body and covers the same amount of our planet. The intent of your words and the words you use can profoundly affect your health and wellbeing.

In the world of Quantum Physics, the deeper the exploration beneath atoms and molecules (the subatomic level), the less substance the body has. Invisible forces, fields and particles, whose interactions underlie not just the human body but all of matter, seem to be at play. This is just the tip of the iceberg with new and extraordinary research coming to light every day.

CHANGE YOUR THOUGHTS; CHANGE YOUR LIFE

When you change your thoughts, your feelings, your behaviours and actions, you can change your material circumstances.

Dr Amen, of The Brain Clinic, has shown that by changing our thought processes in a positive way, we can affect our brain positively too. Although to many people, thoughts, beliefs and hopes are intangibles, you have no doubt heard of someone who healed him or herself with the power of belief, using the power of their mind?

You have probably heard of the placebo effect? Typically, a person getting a placebo – a substance that looks like a medicine, but is not – does not know for sure that the treatment is not real. Even though the placebo does not act on the disease, they tend to have an affect on people's results.

Based on what we have learned about the placebo effect, the way we think and feel about medical treatments can dramatically influence how our bodies respond. It is our belief that is important to our healing.

A *New Scientist* article titled 'Heal thyself' (Ed: 2827, August 2011) stated that for a wide range of conditions, from depression to Parkinson's, osteoarthritis and multiple sclerosis, it is clear that the placebo response is far from imaginary. Trials have shown measurable changes, depending on the beliefs of the patients.

Self-belief is a powerful tool in making change.

Every day I witness the power of belief in my work: my belief and my clients' belief. This is why I feel so privileged to do what I do.

I have worked with a client who eliminated a large cyst in her body after a session helping her release some old emotions or energy that was trapped in her body. (She also embarked on a strict raw food diet.)

I have seen clients let go of nightmares and phobias they have had for 20 years, finding freedom from these debilitating fears. Using specific processes during their session, backed by their desire to change and my belief in the power of the processes, magic has literally happened.

I have helped people break habits of a lifetime and give up cigarettes and alcohol.

I have seen many clients grow in self-esteem and confidence, transforming from being shy to becoming outgoing and powerful.

I have seen clients find the courage to leave dead end jobs and to successfully follow their passion.

I have seen clients break free from toxic relationships, liberate themselves and transform their lives.

I have helped people get out of their rut, back into exercise and transform themselves into 'weekend warriors', doing competitions, fun runs, Ironman Triathlons, mountain climbing and other adventures!

I have worked with business owners, managers and executives who all shared an abiding fear of public speaking. I have seen them overcome their fear, step up and shine.

I have helped procrastinators become massive action takers!

These outcomes occurred because these people were willing to look inside themselves, have the courage to confront their fears and let go of their old patterns. They were willing to believe and to make some changes, take small steps and commit to using the mind tools taught to them.

Yet I know that many people (e.g. the 92% we mentioned before) still don't achieve what they want, because at some level they find it hard to change. The dieters who put on more weight than before... the unused gym memberships... and the books bought with good intention that sit unused on bookshelves. Our programming helps us to avoid 'danger', yet danger represents change. So it seems that we need to work hard to keep the odds in our favour.

Humans are creatures of habit; we are hard-wired to be kept safe and we generally prefer the easy, more comfortable option. We prefer pleasure over pain or instant gratification over long term gain. This is why so many people never achieve what they want. It just seems too hard!

What would happen if you could get outstanding results in your life by reading this book, embracing the learnings and acting upon them? What would that be worth to you? What do you want to change in your life? What do you want to create?

TIME FOR ACTION:

Create a picture in your mind of how your life would be if you had the results you desire. If you can imagine it you can create it, so start working on creating as clear a picture as you can.

Dream big and push yourself beyond your current limitations of what you think is possible. Take a few moments to write down what this picture of your ideal life looks like.

Hopefully you are a bit excited by the possibilities that lie ahead?

WHY CHANGE?

A DECISION IS ALL YOU NEED TO GET STARTED.

'In times of change Learners will inherit the earth; while the Learned find themselves beautifully equipped to deal with a world that no longer exists'.

~ Eric Hoffer

The quote above is one of my favourites. It means if you don't change and evolve, you are either stagnating or dying. That's a truth! It's also important to know that you are the only one who can change yourself. No one else can make you. Not me, not this book, not a magic wand, your partner, friend, spouse, or a course. The knowledge and steps necessary are in this book, but without action, results don't happen.

So, it's time to move out of your comfort zone, knowing that you have to get a little uncomfortable first in order to change. This chapter is all about you taking some action. So, put your thinking cap on and get out your pen and paper.

WHY DO YOU WANT TO CHANGE?

Earlier, I asked you a few questions about what you wanted to change. The next question to ask yourself is:

Why do you want to change? Most people never get crystal clear as to why they want to change.

This is why so many people don't even get started or give up when the going gets tough.

If you already know why you want to change but haven't taken any action towards changing, then there may be an unconscious or conscious belief holding you back, keeping you a prisoner to your current habits and behaviours. Sometimes, there is a benefit for not changing. In Neuro-Linguistic Programming we call it 'secondary gain'. Did you know that some people actually want to remain in their victim mode, sick mode or unhappy mode, because there is a benefit, such as being looked after, feeling safe or protected? The fear of change and fear of losing this benefit keeps them a prisoner to their circumstances. Other people are simply stuck living an uncomfortable, comfortable life. Because we are creatures of habit it often feels easier to live in this comfort zone, even though it may not be fulfilling or even comfortable!

Check in and be honest with yourself. Ask yourself why you want to change. Get crystal clear. It's your why that will help you push over the bumps along the way.

WHAT DO YOU WANT TO CHANGE?

TIME FOR ACTION:

Whether or not you know specifically what you want to change, take a few moments and answer the following questions.

Do you wake up most days feeling happy and content?

Is your life one of your choosing or are you living by someone else's rules?

Are you doing the same thing over and over again and getting the same unwanted results?

How is your health?

What about your food, drink and exercise habits? Do you nurture and look after your body and fuel it for optimal performance?

How are your relationships?

What about your career? Do you love what you do?

Do you easily manage your stress levels, or are you constantly feeling stressed?

If money was not an issue what would you be doing for your vocation? What else would you be doing for yourself?

Reflecting on what you wrote down and what you wrote earlier, write down the area of your life that requires the most attention right now.

Is it your finances, family, relationships or your health? Is it in the area of personal growth or your vocation?

Great! You now have one area to focus on.

WHAT DRIVES YOU TO CHANGE THIS AREA OF YOUR LIFE AND WHO DO YOU WANT TO BE?

> Answer the questions below to get your juices flowing.

> What do you love to do in your life?

> What drives you and inspires you?

> What did you love to do when you were young?

> How do you like to spend your downtime?

> Where would you love to live?

> Who is there with you and what are you doing?

> What sort of person are you now that you have changed?

That should have got the juices flowing. Congratulate yourself for doing this. Now, it's time to continue working on your master change plan.

TIME FOR ACTION:

Compose a few sentences on who you want to become when you have changed.

What will you be doing in your life?

What healthy habits and pursuits will you be doing?

What will you be saying to yourself and what traits will you have embraced in your life?

Is it discipline, focus, enthusiasm, persistence or consistency?

Add these into the picture you created earlier.

Does this add more fuel or excitement to your vision?

Does it make it brighter, bolder or richer? Has it changed the picture?

What is it that's preventing you from achieving your goal?

Now that you have an idea of what you want to change first and what you want to create, let's look at why you haven't already got it.

TIME FOR ACTION:

Write down the answers to these questions. Be honest. Find a quiet place and listen to the answers that come up from that quiet voice deep within.

Is it too hard?

Is it because you didn't have enough time (other priorities)?

Are you not committed?

Do you let other distractions pull you off course?

Do you tend to do things for others and forget about yourself?

Do you blame other people for your circumstances?

Do you think you lack willpower, commitment or resources?

What about the current economic climate or political situation? Do you use these as your excuses or reasons for not being as successful as you want to be?

What else is preventing you from achieving what you want?

Did you uncover anything interesting?
Did you see any patterns or themes emerging?

Congratulations, you have begun to stir things up. Like digging the soil in the garden and bringing weeds to the surface, you are stirring up the subconscious mind. The subconscious is the storehouse of all your memories and experiences and when you stir it up, you are shining light on previously hidden patterns. Getting underneath your layers of protection and becoming aware is vital. Awareness is a key step in making change and creating your master change plan.

As William James, the father of Modern Psychology said:

'The greatest revolution of our generation is the discovery that human beings, by changing the inner

attitudes of their minds, can change the outer aspects of their lives.'

In summary, the clearer you are as to:

> What you want and why you want it, and

> Who you want to be.

The easier it will be to get started and to stay on track when you run into an obstacle.

> **'When you change the way you look at things,
> the things you look at change!'**
> ~ Wayne Dyer

If you want to earn more money, ask yourself why you want to earn money. What will this money give you? Keep asking this question until you get down to the source. It will inevitably be a feeling. If you want better health, get clear as to why you want better health. Why will this benefit your life? What will you be able to do and what will you feel when you have better health? Keep exploring this as you practise the art of asking yourself better questions. Remember to change all statements about what you don't want to what you do want.

Ultimately what you want will be something like fun, freedom, joy or happiness.

GETTING GOING

SETTING YOUR FOCUS - READY, AIM, FIRE!

'Your life only begins to become a great life when you clearly identify what it is that you want, make a plan to achieve it and then work on that plan every single day.'

~ Brian Tracy

You now have an idea of what you want to change, why you want to change, who you want to be and what you want by changing. Like a business wanting to double its profit you need to take out your master plan, your vision, set some goals and act upon them. You need to know where you are headed and what you are aiming at.

WHY IS GOAL SETTING IMPORTANT?

Goal setting is important because you need a focus to keep yourself motivated and inspired and to give you direction in this ever-changing world. Your brain loves to have something to focus on. Setting goals is a way to enable you to bring about the results you want.

If you don't have something to aim for, then you won't know where you are going, why or how.

You may end up like Alice in Lewis Carroll's *Alice in Wonderland*.

> › ALICE: 'I was just wondering... which way should I go?'

> › CAT: 'Well that depends on where you want to be.'

> › ALICE. 'It doesn't really matter.'

> › CAT: 'Well, then it doesn't really matter which way you go.'

A goal gives you a clear target to focus on and aim for. It helps keep you from wandering off the path and getting lost in the big wide world.

Many personal development gurus have cited the importance of goal setting – note the quote above by Brian Tracy. Like me, you may have heard about the often-cited 1953 research study at Yale University, which concluded that the 3% of students who wrote their goals down, when interviewed ten years later, were worth more financially than all the other students? If you Google this study you will see conflicting reports stating that this research was never undertaken! Whether it was or not, I believe it does not negate the importance of setting goals and having clear targets to aim for. If you ask any successful person about their journey, you will find they had a goal, a vision and could clearly articulate their vision to others.

So, in my view, goals are important. Yet it is also important to enjoy the journey along the way and not make the destination (the goals), the be-all and end-all.

POWER TIP.

If the idea of creating and writing goals stresses you out or activates your internal saboteurs, simply rename them. Don't call them goals. Instead, decide to give yourself some gifts or set targets on the road to your success! Use whatever works for you, but please, do set targets for yourself! For simplicity purposes, I will call them goals.

TIME FOR ACTION:

Here are a few questions for you to answer:

Do you have goals?

Do you write them down?

Are they specific and clear?

If you do write goals, when was the last time you reviewed them?

Are you okay with needing to be flexible and changing course if required?

Do you usually achieve your goals?

START SMALL

If you have never set goals, start small. Otherwise you risk never getting started, or giving up very soon into the journey. If you regularly set goals and achieve them, push yourself and set bigger goals. Dare to dream bigger!

Most people underestimate what they can do in the long term and overestimate what they can do in the short term.

As Confucius said, 'It is far better to light one small candle, than to curse the darkness forever.'

Start with small steps, yet dream big!

YOUR LIFE IN 12 MONTHS

TIME FOR ACTION:

Earlier you started to create a picture of your ideal life. Now, let's be more specific.

What do you want your life to look like in 12 months' time?

Imagine there are no limits to what you can do. You can do, be and have whatever you want. You have all the resources you need - people, friends, education, time, money and experience - to accomplish any goal you set for yourself. Wave a magic wand and start imagining. Consider different areas of your life: finances, family, relationships, health, personal growth and contribution. How has this picture evolved or changed from your original one? Is it different, more detailed and specific, or is it similar? Remember, what you can imagine you can create, so the more you spend time creating what you want, the greater your chances of success.

Write down your three most important goals right now. They may be in the area of your life you selected earlier, or in different areas. You choose whatever are the most important goals for you now.

Do this quickly without too much thinking, as often you push down what is really the most important thing. Quick, before your logical brain starts doubting and second-guessing!

TIME FOR ACTION:

Now check each goal in the context of the following questions:

Why do I want this goal?

Does this goal inspire me?

When do I want this by?

Do I believe this is possible?

What or who do I need to help me achieve this goal?

How will I know when I have achieved this goal?

What will I be seeing, hearing and feeling to know it is real for me?

Write down the answers to the questions. Note how you feel when you do this.

Take a moment to congratulate yourself for taking action and getting started.

CRAFTING YOUR GOALS

You now have some goals and hopefully, they should excite you!

The next step is to craft your goals and set a clear target to focus on. It's much easier to hit a target you can see, isn't it?

Your goals need to be short, clearly written and written in the present tense (as if now).

Your goals need to have a specific date you want to achieve them by.

It is critically important to engage yourself fully in the goal. To imagine how you will be feeling in the moment you have achieved it. As Neville says, *'standing in the moment of the wish fulfilled'*. Step into your goal and notice everything that is happening in full sensory detail, especially how you feel.

HOW TO SUCCINCTLY WRITE YOUR GOALS

> 'It is now 01 December 2015 and I have just completed my first half marathon and I am feeling so excited, happy and proud.'

Clarity creates focus and gives you energy in the pursuit of your goals. The more clarity and excitement you have, the more you will create a laser-like focus and the quicker the arrow can hit the bulls-eye. Your goals must be realistic to you and excite you. Otherwise you will probably give up. Write your goals in the present tense with a specific date on them, such as 01 December 2015. Get engaged in the defining moment of achievement. Imagine taking a snapshot of this moment of your success. Step into this moment and imagine living it right now.

As you stand in that moment, what will you be doing, seeing, hearing, feeling or knowing when you have achieved your goal? Imagine feeling the feeling of being right there right now. I call this the 'end' step. It is a critical component in the creation of your goals. It helps you lock it into your subconscious mind.

HERE ARE A FEW GROUND RULES FOR CREATING AND ACHIEVING YOUR GOALS:

> Set clear and realistic goals.

> Act on your goals.

> Take small steps daily.

> Review and revise your goals when required.

> Always keep your goal at the front of your mind!

> Be clear about why you want your goals.

> Write your goals in present time.

TIME FOR ACTION:

Write out all your goals in the above format.

Awesome! You now have some goals, targets with deadlines! For each goal, write down a summary of the steps required to achieve it. Consider this in the context of who you may need to help you, the obstacles you may encounter and the action steps required. The more steps you can identify, the easier it will be for your brain to start focussing on what needs to be done, rather than focussing on how on earth you can achieve your goal?

Next, you can set smaller targets and deadlines within the larger goal. You need deadlines to help you achieve them, like plotting your progress on a map when driving from Cairns to Sydney, by marking off the towns you pass along the way.

Detailed action plans and lists give the brain something to focus on. It is also the antidote to overwhelm, panic and procrastination!

Now you need to keep focussed on the most important thing to do. Write down the following sentence on a piece of paper.

*'What is the most important thing
for me to do right now?'*

Put this on your desk or in a prominent place, for times when you have lost focus, have been pulled off course, or don't know what to do next.

Remember, if you aim at nothing, you are bound to hit it!

*Remember to set yourself rewards, find
someone to keep you accountable and keep
plugged into the big reason you want this goal.*

This is why successful people have coaches to help them stay on track.

Brian Tracy, an expert on human behaviour and achievement, has more to say about setting goals:

'No other quality, such as environment, appearance, grade level or family background, is nearly as important to personal success as the habit of personal goal-setting. It is intense goal-orientation that marks the winners in every single area. Unless we have goals, we simply go around in circles in our lives. We go nowhere.'

Congratulations. You now have a master plan with goals and your first action steps. At best you will have detailed a number of steps for each goal. If you are feeling overwhelmed, keep it simple. Pick one goal and start with the first action step required. If your goal is to get fitter and lose some weight, choose one task (say of walking twice a week) and stick to doing it for at least 30 days. Make it a ritual and do it! Stick with your ritual and it will become a habit.

Getting started, persistence and consistency are important in creating new habits.

WANT FURTHER HELP WITH GOAL SETTING?

There is an entire module dedicated to goal setting in my online course, available from my website: **www.mindsetforsuccess.com.au/90-day-online-coaching/**.

You will learn how to craft your goals, as well as:

> How to send your goal into the Universe (including an audio process).

> A hypnosis audio to help you stay on track.

> BONUS module to help you plan your best year yet. This outlines a detailed and precise system for planning your year in a very specific manner and how to test and measure your progress to keep moving forward.

When you use the **Powerful Mind Tools** featured in this course, you will become unstoppable!

Success is created by the sum total of daily disciplines. Success is created by small steps repeated daily, consistently, over a lifetime.

INSIDE YOUR AMAZING MIND

YOUR MIND CONSISTS OF TWO PARTS

'If you correct your mind, the rest of your life will fall into place.'

~ Lao-tze

Before we go further, I want to take you deeper into the mind, to help you understand and learn a bit more about this incredible organ you have between your ears!

Your mind is your driving force, or perhaps the connection between you and what you experience in your outer world.

One definition of the word Mind from the Merriam-Webster dictionary is:

'The element or complex of elements in an individual that feels, perceives, thinks, wills and especially reasons.'

You have probably heard that our minds consist of two parts, the **Conscious Mind** (sometimes referred to as the Rational or Logical Mind) and the **Unconscious** or **Subconscious mind**. Throughout this book I will refer to this part of the mind as the Subconscious mind, as it is the part that lies beneath the surface. It is also referred to as the Unconscious Mind, because this is what Milton Erickson, probably the greatest Hypnotist of all times, called it. He was responsible for the acceptance of hypnosis as a modality in the Medical world.

It is commonly recognised that we only use around ten percent of our potential, which represents our Conscious Mind. Studies undertaken at Stanford University's Brain Institute show that it is probably closer to only two percent. So we really do have an abundance of unknown possibilities and unused abilities. Our Subconscious Mind constitutes around ninety percent of our mind, is way more powerful than our conscious mind and the reason you need to learn to work with it to get the results you desire. Both parts of the mind have separate, differing functions.

The Conscious Mind is where we do all our logical thinking and is the part of the mind where we make our choices. It is sometimes referred to as our objective mind, because it deals with outward objects. It is aware of the world outside of us and it processes information by way of our five physical senses: sight, sound, touch, taste and smell. It is also where our willpower is.

Our Conscious Mind learns through observation, experience and education. Its greatest function is its reasoning. Picture yourself travelling overseas and visiting the Taj Mahal in India. You would probably conclude that it is one of the wonders of the world, based on your observations of the incredible mosaics, the structure, components and sheer size and beauty of the building. You would marvel at the way the colours change in the marble and compare it to your preconceived ideas. This is how the Conscious mind works. It observes, experiences, compares, contrasts and makes logical decisions.

Our Subconscious mind is the part that runs our lives. Without any conscious thought or effort, it keeps our heart functioning, it keeps all of our vital functions going – such as our circulation, digestion and breathing – as we get on with the job of living. It has no logical or analytical processes. It is subjective and just accepts what is impressed upon it every day. It never engages in what is good or bad, even though its primary function is to protect us.

The subconscious mind acts upon and according to what it is fed; what thoughts, pictures, sounds or words it is given.

It is the seat of all our emotions and the storehouse of our memories. It is also the domain of perhaps our most powerful tool, our imagination.

'Imagination is more important than knowledge.'
~ Einstein

'Imagination rules the world.'
~ Disraeli

'The greatest achievement was at first and for a time a dream. The oak sleeps in the acorn; the bird waits in the egg; and in the highest vision of the soul a waking angel stirs. Dreams are the seedlings of realities.'
~ James Allen

The Subconscious mind is where our habits are stored and where all learning, change and behaviour firstly take place.

With all these attributes, to create lasting change, it is imperative to work in this deep, subconscious mind in order to ensure both parts of the mind work together (and not in opposition).

The law of the mind goes like this:

'The reaction or response you get from your subconscious mind will be determined by the nature of the thought or idea you hold in your conscious mind.'

Our subconscious mind performs at its highest function when our objective senses are not functioning. It is functioning when you arrive at your destination and know you drove safely but can't really recall getting there. It is functioning in the classic 'flight or fight response' and is also in charge when you had all good intentions to eat healthily yet at the end of the day you succumbed to your usual evening hot chocolate, pulling out a habitual program because you 'forgot' to use your conscious mind to make a herbal tea instead.

Your habitual actions and thinking establishes deep grooves in the subconscious mind.

Turning to bad foods at particular times of the day creates a habit, a habit that we can feel powerless to change. Once an idea is accepted, your subconscious begins to execute it, whether it's a good or bad idea.

To explain the power of our Subconscious mind in another way, imagine your Conscious mind is the Captain of a ship and the Subconscious mind is the crew. Even though the Captain gives the orders because she is in charge, it's the crew who run the ship. They are the ones doing the work, stoking the boiler room, checking the gauges and instruments. If the crew don't follow the Captain's orders, mutiny can occur!

In life, many people have mutiny within their minds. All our beliefs, emotions, habits and memories are stored in our subconscious mind and too often, they show up as inner conflicts or self-sabotaging patterns. These conflicts or patterns create unfulfilled goals and inconsistent results.

Consider a time when you might have had mutiny in your life. How many New Year's Resolutions have you made and then given up on? Have you started an exercise regime and let it fall by the wayside, or started a project that never came to fruition? Most likely I think!

Just like a farmer who sows seeds (our thoughts) into a fertile soil (subconscious mind), the mind will sprout whatever thoughts are sown. Seeds of thistles will sprout thistles… and seeds of roses will sprout roses! In life we make time to clean the house, wash our clothes and tidy our desk. Sometimes we take care of our body with a massage. Yet why do so few people invest in a mind, life or business coach? A mindset or life coach can help you 'spring clean' and create room for new ideas; they support and guide you on your journey through the complexities of life to achieve great results.

Over the past years, I have helped many smokers become non-smokers. The majority of these people had tried some other method to quit. A few tried it with their 'willpower', while others gave patches or a medically prescribed drug a try. Prior to seeing me, most believed it was hard to quit.

There are a few people who quit 'just like that'. They made a decisive decision and gave a clear instruction to their subconscious mind with conviction (total belief) and hey presto, like magic, it worked. No side effects, cravings or withdrawals transpired. These people though, are in the minority. That is why hypnosis and the tools and techniques within the spectrum of Neuro-Linguistic Programming are so powerful with helping people to change habits. They are focussing on the subconscious, the home of our habits.

Can you picture an iceberg? Most of it lies beneath the surface.

This is rather like your mind. The top of the iceberg, above the water, is your conscious mind. The larger, hidden, yet powerful area below is your subconscious mind.

Every one of your conscious thoughts contributes to the building of your subconscious mind. When you learned to eat using a knife and fork, it took much conscious thought and effort. When you learned to drive, it took an immense amount of conscious effort. Over time, your deftness with your knife and fork became a part of your subconscious programming, a habit, so that now you rarely miss your mouth! You can probably drive with ease and quite often aren't even aware of how you arrived at your destination. Again, your subconscious mind has created a habit.

WHY IS THE SUBCONSCIOUS SO POWERFUL?

In the book *The Magic of Believing*, Claude Bristol stated, 'Just as the conscious mind is the source of thought, so the subconscious is the source of power.' Your subconscious mind contains your programs for walking, talking, solving problems when you are asleep, healing your body, saving your life in times of danger and much more. It contains the sum total of all your conscious thoughts up until this very moment.

Whatever you have deposited into your subconscious mind by way of your day-to-day thoughts is now producing the results in your life.

Becoming aware of your actions and ensuring your thoughts are in alignment with what you want is a vital step to changing your results. Your thoughts are the currency of your results.

I have purposely elaborated on the subconscious mind, because the key to your success is to make friends with this amazing part of your mind and harness your magnificent powers inside.

Remember, that your mind always tries to complete what it pictures. The more strongly you can visualise what you want and feel the excitement of getting what you want, the more powerfully you will attract what you want.

What have you been programming your subconscious mind with? If you aren't sure, take a look at the results you have in your life today.

Program your subconscious mind constantly with what you want. Recognise when you are acting out an old program that could be sabotaging your success. Be conscious of your thoughts and responsible for your actions.

HOW DO YOU VIEW YOUR LIFE?

SEEING IS BELIEVING... OR IS IT?

'The human being is born with his perception already somewhat obscured and he harms himself even more by denying, distorting or omitting reality.'

~ Norberto R. Keppe

It has been postulated in the field of Neuroscience that our nervous systems are bombarded with two million bits of information every second. Imagine being exposed to at least two million bits of information every second, absorbed by your five senses: sight, sound, touch, sense, taste and smell. To prevent overload of information, you must delete, distort and generalise it to make sense of it. You filter this information down to the amount that your conscious mind can handle at any one time, around seven plus or minus two 'chunks' of information.

In life you are creating your own version of what is real by making meaning out of your experiences.

When you distil two million bits to only one hundred and thirty-six bits (seven plus or minus two), do you think you might be limiting your perspective in life? It is what we delete, distort and generalise that causes us to 'see' what we view in the world. We put a meaning on this experience and it becomes our truth or reality.

The filters we use to process this vast amount of information are unique to every individual. Our filters were created when we were young. They consist of our beliefs, our values, our attitudes, memories, emotions, language and how we view the world. They were shaped by our experiences from the environment we were raised in, the people we modelled or spent time with (often our parents, family and teachers) and any other significant events that occurred when we were young. This is why many people can experience the same event yet have a totally different perspective or version of the event. It has been said that in the imprint period, from around nought to seven years old, most of our beliefs are formed.

Many of our beliefs were literally 'imprinted' in us without our conscious awareness.

Think of a few generic statements you may have heard when you were young. Phrases like: 'Money doesn't grow on trees', 'Money is the root of all evil', or 'Children should be seen and not heard.' Or like my client Susan, 'You must finish the food on your plate'.

While we can't change the past, when we become conscious of the beliefs that we view the world with, we can begin to dismantle their hold over us, if they do not serve us. Releasing them expands our possibilities, allows us to see things differently and to choose a new way of thinking and behaving in life, giving us different results.

We have billions of unused connections in our mind and body, equating to more potential than we could ever use in our lifetime.

Every time you expand your thinking, come up with a new idea, or see something from a new perspective, options and possibilities open up for you. So, actions, behaviours and results will change.

To help you expand your thinking, use questions that expand possibilities. When you ask yourself a question starting with 'how', it presupposes possibilities. Your mind does not like unanswered questions, so it seeks to find a solution, thus opening yourself up to creativity and curiosity.

What you focus or concentrate on, you will bring into your reality.

If your focus is on how hard it is to change, or what a terrible upbringing you had, or how hard life is, all you are doing is locking these thought patterns in. Thoughts and feelings attract similar thoughts and feelings. The universe is a mirror of what is going on in the inside and what you project out into the external world. It will reflect back whatever you project out.

TIME FOR ACTION:

What do you consistently think about?

Do you focus on what you want or what you don't want?

Do you tend to be optimistic or pessimistic?

How would your results change if you practised focussing on what you want and you trained yourself to think positively?

TAKE RESPONSIBILITY

YOUR CHOICES COUNT

'The difference between a successful person and others, is not a lack of strength, not a lack of knowledge, but rather a lack of will.'
~ Vince Lombardi

In Neuro-Linguistic Programming (NLP), one of the presuppositions is that of **Cause and Effect**. We have a choice every day to live 'at cause', where we take responsibility for our lives, or to live 'at effect', where we blame others.

If we live at cause and take full responsibility, we accept that we are in control of our actions. When we realise we are responsible for the consequences of those actions, even if they are not as we had anticipated, we can take stock, accept, learn and re-evaluate our next steps to change the results we are getting.

If we choose to live life at the effect side, we believe that things happen to us and we have no control over the outcomes. In other words, we blame things, people, places or situations outside of ourselves for why things didn't work out. Consider how often you hear people blaming others, the economy, the weather, the government, their partner or spouse?

WHAT OR WHO DO YOU BLAME WHEN THINGS DON'T GO YOUR WAY?

Do you do this? How often? If you do, then at some level you have chosen to believe that you are powerless over your life, your thoughts, your emotions and that life just 'happens'.

If you are living your life on the side of effect, ask yourself how your results would change if you chose to live life on the side of cause?

The acceptance of personal responsibility is fundamental to achieve great success in life.

TIME FOR ACTION:

If you aren't already taking full responsibility for every aspect of your life, I challenge you to do this.

Pretend for a day that you are totally responsible for everything that occurs to you in your life.

Do it for another day, then a week and then a month.

Do it until it becomes a habit and a way of life.

Commit to accepting ultimate responsibility for every aspect of your life and see how your results change.

Be conscious of your actions and responsible for your choices.

WHAT DO YOU BELIEVE?

ARE YOUR BELIEFS SABOTAGING YOUR LIFE?

'If you don't change your beliefs, your life will be like this forever. Is that good news?'
~ W. Somerset Maugham

A belief is: *a statement that you say to yourself about something you assume to be true.* Beliefs help you cement understanding of the world you live in. They can be empowering or limiting. Over time, your beliefs become entrenched statements of fact that you view your life through. Effectively, they become your reality.

As I mentioned earlier, beliefs are usually created early on in life, during the formative years up to the age of about seven. This period is when information is more easily absorbed without much discernment. Influential people at this time – parents, teachers and family members – knowingly or unknowingly pass on their own beliefs and values. These beliefs eventually become an ingrained set of statements operating at the subconscious level, usually beneath the level of conscious awareness. They exert tremendous impact on people's identity, both in a positive and a negative manner.

Beliefs are like deep grooves,
programs that direct lives in unconscious ways
as to how things should be, could be or are
supposed to be.

Your life experiences will be reflected in different areas of your life depending on your beliefs.

If you don't believe that you can change, you won't. If you don't believe you can heal, you won't. It is imperative you work towards a total belief in yourself. If you don't believe in yourself, how can you expect anyone else too?

Limiting beliefs, especially the ones that have been programmed into you since you were young will show up in your life in all areas. They can mar and sabotage your relationships, wealth, health, career, happiness and opportunities.

LIMITING BELIEFS

HERE ARE A FEW EXAMPLES OF LIMITING AND POTENTIALLY
SABOTAGING BELIEFS:

> 'Money doesn't grow on trees.'

> 'Money is the root of all evil.'

> 'The world is a dangerous place.'

> 'What you fear makes you stronger.'

> 'Life is never fair.'

> 'You must work hard to earn money.'

> 'Finish your plate. Think of the poor starving
  people in the world.'

> 'Children should be seen and not heard.'

Imagine how these beliefs could influence someone's life. What a different life someone would lead if they believed the world was a dangerous place, compared to someone who believed the world was a safe place. What about someone who believes it's hard to earn money compared to someone who believes opportunities are everywhere? Do you see how this could potentially limit or even sabotage their success in work and income opportunities?

The first step is to become aware of all of your beliefs... the good, bad and the indifferent.

TIME FOR ACTION:

Take some time to write down as many beliefs as you can remember being told when you were young. Highlight the ones that may have limited you in your life.

TIP:

If you don't have the level of wealth, health, happiness or relationships that you desire, you will definitely have limiting beliefs! Consider how they may have shaped your decisions in your life.

Now answer the questions below to help you uncover more limiting beliefs, as these will be limiting the results you desire in some form.

What are you lacking in your life? Consider this in all areas: Money, savings, health, relationships, opportunities, social, fun, adventure, travel, happiness.

What excuses are you making when it comes to why you lack what you do?

Do you have any idea why you are making these excuses?

Are you generally a positive or pessimistic person and why do you think this is?

What makes you angry?

What do you most fear?

Are you a perfectionist in all or some areas of your life and how is this perhaps holding you back or causing you stress?

What do you find yourself settling for or giving in to?

When you look in the mirror, what do you normally say to yourself?

How much doubt do you have about achieving what you want in your life?

I doubt myself because...?

Did you answer these questions honestly?

Congratulations for doing this! Now highlight every belief, statement or word that may be limiting your life.

*Your beliefs are directly responsible for your
current results.*

Mentally read each belief. Gauge how they make you feel and what pictures, feelings, sounds or self-talk each belief brings up for you. Remember you do not have to be defined by your beliefs. You may have unconsciously adopted them at a time when you were too young to question their validity.

Before Roger Bannister broke the four-minute mile, no one believed it was possible. It was thought the heart would explode at that speed and Roger's coach didn't even believe he could do it! When Roger Bannister broke this milestone, the belief was shattered and many runners soon achieved even faster times. Once upon a time, it was thought that the world was flat and people would have laughed at the possibility of flying to the moon. What else can you think of that has occurred and once was thought to be impossible?

I point these things out so that you understand you can transform your limiting beliefs. Don't let them define your life. Commit to questioning all of your long held assumptions.

TIME FOR ACTION

Questions to change limiting beliefs:

Take each belief and run them through the following questions. Set a clear Intention to come up with a new meaning that would splinter the old belief into two.

Where did you learn this from?

Is this true for every person in the world?

Do you really believe it?

How do you feel and react when you think of this belief?

What has this belief cost you?

What has it prevented you from doing, having or being?

What results could occur if you could let go of this belief?

How do you feel when you consider these results?

Could you now make a new belief and adopt it, try it out?

How does that new belief feel?

Write out a list of your new beliefs and practise saying them to yourself until you truly believe them.

Clearing beliefs is a critical step in making long-term changes.

Once upon a time, the top people in every field were not in that field. At one point, they didn't even know it existed. Current Olympic gold medallists were once not-so-good at their sport and many didn't even know they could be a master at it before they gave it a go and focussed on it!

If countless others can change and become good at something they once knew nothing about, or were not good at, you can too! It really comes down to the starting blocks, i.e. making a decision to get going and to build your belief in yourself.

If you currently don't fully believe in yourself, a great way to build your belief is to create a statement such as 'Every day I am becoming more confident'. Then imagine yourself being a bit more confident every day. If you do this consistently you will soon build your self-belief.

WATCH YOUR LANGUAGE!

SAY IT HOW YOU REALLY WANT IT TO BE

'We are what we think. All that we are arises with our thoughts. With our thoughts we make the world. Speak or act with a pure mind and happiness will follow you as your shadow unshakeable.'

~ The Dhammapada

Now you have created some goals and made a start uncovering your beliefs, it's time to introduce a few fundamental starting tools necessary to help you create healthier, positive habits.

Why your thoughts and self-talk are vital keys to creating change.

Whatever you habitually think about inevitably comes about. Your thoughts stem from your beliefs and show up in your life in your results. One of the most powerful ways to change your results is to become aware of your thoughts. Your habitual thoughts become your attitude, so if you want to become more positive about your life, change your thoughts!

If you are repeatedly thinking about what you don't want, or you are beating yourself up for not getting the results you expect, all you are doing is poisoning your mind and body and ensuring you get what you don't want!

Imagine if what you said to yourself showed up in a bubble above your head for everyone to see. Would you then be more careful about what you say to yourself?

As we mentioned before, all matter – including us humans – is made up of energy and everything is connected. So, if we are energy and all connected, what we think and feel will be reflected out from us and in some way, reflected back. As our mind and body are inextricably connected, that means our subconscious mind – the reservoir of all our habits, unresolved emotions, memories and past 'stuff' – is part of our entire body. This is the reason that our negative self-talk and emotions can and do manifest as physical ailments or 'dis-ease' within our body.

Your subconscious mind cannot process
negatives directly.

When you say, 'I mustn't have that piece of chocolate cake,' or, 'I can't get that job as I don't have enough experience,' you are effectively feeding it what you don't want. And remember, what you focus on in life is what you create.

Your subconscious mind grabs onto key words, words with an emotional charge or imagery. For it to compute not having chocolate cake, it focuses on the very thing you are trying to not focus on, chocolate cake. That is one reason why many people fail to create and maintain healthy habits.

They spend their time focussing on what they don't want, whether it be trying not to think about eating, drinking, smoking, or not wanting to be broke, or worrying about not being good enough to stand up and speak. If you don't take control of your imagination, it takes control over you… and it will win over willpower anytime!

Perhaps this is how you have been operating in your life? If so, does it help explain why you haven't created the results you desire yet?

The more you become congruent with what you are thinking, feeling, saying and seeing, the clearer your message will be sent out to the receivers in the Universe and the more of the good stuff you will get back! Positive statements about yourself and what you want in life will help you create just that. In the words of Norman Vincent Peale, 'You are not what you think you are... but what you think, you are.'

TIME FOR ACTION

Write out a mantra or positive statement that will help you become the new you.

If you wrote one out from the work you did on your beliefs, great. If not, take a few moments and do it now.

Here are a few examples for you:

'Every day I am becoming even more confident and empowered.'

'It is easy to focus on fuelling my body with healthy choices.'

'Every day I am becoming healthier and more energetic.'

THE HIDDEN POWER OF YOUR WORDS

If you haven't seen Dr Masaru Emoto's videos on the power of words and water, then find him on YouTube or Google. You can also see this on the documentary *What the Bleep* or read his book called *The Message from Water*. His research demonstrated that human vibrational energy, thoughts, words, ideas and music affect the molecular structure of water. The same water that makes up around 70% of a mature human body and covers the same amount of our planet.

After giving good words to crystals of frozen water, he always observed beautiful crystals and with negative words, the opposite – disfigured crystals.

Imagine what your language could be doing to your results and the health of your body? If your body was a fertile garden that reaps whatever it is sown, are you planting seeds for beautiful fruits to be harvested… or toxic weeds?

THE MAGNETISM OF YOUR MIND

Have you ever been thinking of someone you haven't seen in months and suddenly they call you or you run into them in the street? Have you ever been singing an old song to yourself and then you suddenly heard it playing on the radio? What about if you found yourself living in the place that you had imagined living in years before, the street or even house?

People often group such occurrences under the label of 'coincidence', but I believe there is something greater at work here. Your mind is a magnet and you attract what you think about. The same principles of magnetism and attraction that we observe in the 'physical' world are also at work on the invisible plane. If you delve into the thousands of self-help and personal development books, or explore the amazing world of Quantum Physics, this will be shown to you over and over again.

HERE ARE FOUR QUOTES TO ILLUSTRATE THIS:

'Our brains become magnetised with the dominating thoughts which we hold in our minds and, by means with which no man is familiar, these "magnets" attract to us the forces, the people, the circumstances of life which harmonise with the nature of our dominating thoughts.'

~ Napoleon Hill

'A man sooner or later discovers that he is the master-gardener of his soul, the director of his life. He also reveals, within himself, the laws of thought, and understands, with ever increasing accuracy, how the thought-forces and mind elements operate in the shaping of his character, circumstances and destiny.'

~ James Allen, As a Man Thinketh

'Our fear thoughts are just as creative or just as magnetic in attracting troubles to us as the constructive and positive thoughts in attracting positive results. So no matter what the character of the thought it does create after its own kind. ... What may appear as coincidences are not coincidences at all but simply the working out of the pattern which you started with your own weaving.'

~ Claude Bristol, The Magic of Believing

'We magnetise into our lives whatever we hold in our thoughts.'

~ Richard Bach

If radio waves pass easily through wood, brick, steel and other supposedly solid objects, then it is probable that thought vibration can too. If thought waves are turned into even higher oscillations, then they surely can affect the molecules of solid objects. What power, therefore, your thoughts truly hold!

BECOME THE MASTER OF YOUR THOUGHTS

As the Buddhists say, you must learn to 'surf on the waves of your thoughts'. It's a much happier alternative to being tossed and pummelled around in a big ocean! So how can you do this?

Just observe your thoughts as they come and go. Watch them and do not react. Allow your thoughts to rise, just as waves do, but choose to observe and ride them smoothly. Every day, notice when your thoughts start racing and you start to feel stressed. Stop what you are doing and observe what is going on. What are you thinking? Where are the thoughts coming from... your conscious mind or your pre-programmed subconscious mind? What situation is causing them?

The more you learn to detach from these thoughts, the less likely you are to be at their mercy.

TIME FOR ACTION:

When you have practised the art of observing your thoughts, commit to observe what you say to yourself for a period of 30 days. Do this with no judgment. Simply observe.

When you hear yourself talking about what you don't want, simply change the program and state what you want instead. Just like a television, there are many channels running simultaneously. If you are watching the ABC, you don't know what is happening on SBS until you change the channel. If you don't like the TV station you are watching you can change it!

The same applies to your thoughts and self talk. If you don't like your story, change it. You can even imagine saying to yourself, '**Change the channel.**' Add in a step that works for you.

ACTION TIME

TAKE SMALL STEPS CONSISTENTLY

*'Desire is the key to motivation, but
it's determination and commitment to
an unrelenting pursuit of your goal – a
commitment to excellence – that will enable
you to attain the success you seek.'*
~ Mario Andretti

You now have the fundamentals and some tools for getting started with changing. You have explored your beliefs, started to loosen your limiting beliefs and become more aware of the chatter in your head. You have created one or more positive statements to help you change and have a technique to become the master of your thoughts. You have some fundamental mind tools. Now it's time to take some action.

You have probably heard the saying, *'A goal without action is just a dream.'* To ensure you create healthy, positive habits and the results you desire, you must be consistently moving forward, heading in the general direction of what you want. This takes conscious effort and persistence. Until you have well and truly locked the new habits in, you may have a tendency to slip back to old ways... like a rubber band returning to its original size before you stretched it.

Much research has been carried out on the topic of habits, how to give up bad habits and create healthy ones. The reality is, habits are easier to make than they are to break. When you repeat a behaviour often enough, you are literally repeating a pattern that becomes 'worn in' to your brain.

When you wake up, have a cup of coffee, a cigarette, shower, drive to work, buying a cappuccino and muffin for your breakfast, in that order, every morning, the pattern is etched into your brain, in the form of well-used synaptic pathways. It becomes easier for impulses to travel along these pathways and the behaviour seems 'natural'.

TAKE SMALL STEPS AND MAKE RITUALS

To ensure you give yourself the best chance of success, it is best to take small steps consistently. That may mean you need to set small goals to start with, breaking the big goal down to smaller steps.

As we are motivated towards pleasure and away from pain, the thought of giving up all those habits in one go, causes many people to either give up quickly or to not even make an attempt! Although I know exceptional people can change their habits with one decision, the reality is that most people struggle.

In my research on habits, I have read it can take anywhere between 21 to 30 days to change a habit and up to 110 days to lock it in. However, I am not entirely sure where the 21 day rule originated from, but I found it referenced in one of the early self helps books published in the 1970s, a book called *Psycho-Cybernetics*, written by Maxwell Maltz.

Perhaps when you think of doing what is necessary to create healthy habits, you hear that voice telling you, 'It's too hard.' Or, 'Maybe I will start tomorrow.' Perhaps you think you don't have enough willpower. If this is you, consider the idea of creating daily rituals instead. In the book *The Power of Full Engagement*, Jim Loehr and Tony Schwartz suggest that when it comes to change, instead of focussing on cultivating self-discipline as a means toward change, instead focus on introducing rituals. They say, *'Building rituals requires defining very precise behaviours and performing them at very specific times.'* When these are motivated by deeply held values around our identity, it becomes easier to change.

From first-hand knowledge as an athlete, I know athletes value training, being fit and at the top of their game. It is easy for athletes to train because of this value. Likewise, for artists who love to create, they would value taking time to express themselves creatively. When you are motivated by a deeply held value, it is easier to start doing what is needed to create the everyday habits you desire to practise and getting started is good!

TIME FOR ACTION:

Write down what you value in life. A value is what you judge to be important in your life. Values are usually one word or short phrases, such as integrity, fun, adventure, family, sharing, travel, religion, honesty, trust, exercise, being creative.

When you are clear on what you value and your goals are in alignment with your values, it's easier to move towards them. It is also easier to create simple rituals that will become your habits, habits that will help you create the change you desire.

Ask yourself now: 'what one ritual could I add in to my day that would help me create a healthy habit and allow me to create the change I desire?' If you want to start an exercise regime but find it hard to get started, yet you value your family, perhaps you could introduce a ritual of having a family walk at the weekend when you merely get together, run around and have fun. This means you connect as a family while doing some exercise. It may be a great way to start to love exercising and it might help you feel happier too!

Be creative. You are only limited by your imagination. Perhaps you could catch up with a friend and go for a walk or go a gym class together? Would that make it more fun? Pick one small action that feels realistic and doable and excites you just a little bit!

Say you want to cut down on high sugar food and drink. If you set rigid rules and give up everything at once, you risk feeling resentful or rebellious and will probably fail. What one small step could you make a ritual out of? Could you make Mondays a no sugar day, or a fruit and vegetable day? Could you eat from a smaller plate three nights a week? Whatever you choose, pick one thing and commit to this one thing until it becomes a habit.

Action breeds action and makes you feel good.

Warren Buffet said, 'I don't try to jump over seven foot bars, I look around for one foot bars I can step over', while the author Tony Schwartz said, 'incremental change is better than ambitious failure… Success feeds on itself.'

Great advice!

POWER TIP

Keep a Journal of your successes. This will allow you to look back and see how far you have come. Not only will this help you feel good about yourself, it will also help you program your mind to look for the things you usually miss. Most people are good at noting what they didn't do right, not what they did well! Remember, success fuels success.

WHERE IS YOUR FOCUS?

KEEPING YOURSELF FOCUSSED ON WHAT YOU WANT

'You have everything you need.
A miraculous body, a phenomenal brain
and a vast powerful subconscious mind.
Now it's just a matter of focussing them
in the right direction.'
~ James Allen

By now you will realise that it's critical to ensure your language is positive and you become diligent about what you say to yourself. In line with this, it is vitally important to keep focussed on what you want in order to create the success you desire. The more you program yourself to keep focussed on what you want, the more your chance of success.

REMEMBER:

> Your conscious mind has a short-term memory.

> You lose focus around every 6-8 seconds.

> You are hardwired to be kept safe.

> You are a creature of habit.

HERE ARE TWO TECHNIQUES TO HELP YOU KEEP FOCUSSED ON WHAT YOU WANT:

1. Self-programming for success

Your subconscious mind, the 'crew' who follow the captain's instructions (your conscious mind), are great followers, but lousy leaders. They like simple, clear instructions, repeated frequently. When you give yourself clear, positive instructions, you are working your mind muscle and creating a habit of keeping yourself focussed on what you want.

A good time to program yourself is at night, before you go to sleep. When you are in a resting state your subconscious mind, your crew, is more open to suggestions. Self-programming at night is like giving yourself good medicine before you go to sleep. A healthy tonic for the crew to absorb while you sleep, because your subconscious mind never sleeps. It is awake twenty-four seven, even while you sleep!

One way to easily self-program yourself is to listen to a Hypnosis or relaxation audio at night. I have produced a range of Hypnosis Audios as a tool to assist people in making positive changes to their lives. They are available on my website: http://www.mindsetforsuccess.com.au in the products section.

The audios *Ideal Weight* and *Healthy Habits* are tailored to assist with weight loss and the creation of healthy eating and exercise habits. The *Success While You Sleep* audio is designed to help you create your goals and design your ideal life.

Hypnosis has been proven to be a powerful modality to help people make changes in their lives. It is used in many fields from medicine, dentistry, business, sports and therapy. The more you continue embedding your subconscious mind with positive suggestions, the greater the chances are of locking in the changes. As most people sleep between six to eight hours, hypnosis audios are a great tool to use when you are resting before you go to sleep at night.

2. Self-programming to create change

The second way to program yourself is with your own words and statements. Your subconscious mind, which is suggestible, likes to be told things three times, three different ways and simply stated. The suggestion has power when you accept it mentally. Then, your subconscious powers begin to act according to the nature of the suggestion.

If you want to get out of bed at 5.30am and go to the gym, you can easily program yourself to do so. You will be amazed at how successful this can be! Just program yourself before you drift off to sleep, with what you want to happen when you wake up. Say it three times in three slightly different ways. Here is an example:

> 'When the alarm goes off I will wake up feeling alert, full of energy and excited about going to the gym at 5.30am.'

> 'The moment my alarm goes off at 5.30am I will wake up feeling full of energy, ready to jump out of bed and excited to go to the gym.'

> 'The moment I wake up at 5.30am I will get up feeling alive, excited and ready to go to the gym.'

If you do this consistently, you will find yourself waking up just before the alarm goes off, ready to get out of bed, perhaps with a spring in your step!

You can also use this methodology to help you solve a problem. Give yourself clear instructions to resolve the issue before you go to sleep. Say something like: 'When I wake up in the morning I will easily find the answer to my problem.'

You form habits by repeating a thought until it establishes new pathways in the brain. Therefore, you can make up your own mantra and repeat it with belief and conviction throughout the day. If, for instance you want to heal, you could make your own self-healing mantra. You must believe you can heal and have an intention to heal, because a belief in what you want to happen is critical in your success.

You could say something like:

'The healing intelligence of my subconscious mind that created my body is now working towards perfect health. It is healing every cell, nerve, tissue, muscle and organ according to my perfect blueprint of health. Moment by moment, old and redundant thought patterns are being released. Old emotions and stagnant energy is being released and dissolved. My body is becoming increasingly vital and healthy. I am becoming more receptive to easily allowing the innate healing powers of my inner wisdom to heal my body. Every day my body is healing in every way.'

Consider it like a gym workout for the mind. You know that when people consistently go to the gym and lift weights they improve their muscle strength, don't you? If you don't use your muscles, they will wither away. The more you use these simple tools and techniques, the more you are flexing your mind muscle, building it up to create new habits and new programs. When you start to see results, it will spur you on to keep using them.

MIND POWER

DIRECTING YOUR FOCUS...
WITH INTENTIONS

*'Leave the mirror and change your face.
Leave the world alone and change your
conceptions of yourself.'*
~ Neville Goddard

THE POWER OF FOCUS IS A KEY INGREDIENT TO SUCCESS

Imagine for a moment that you have a goal, something that you want to achieve, today, tomorrow or in a week's time. Focus on it fully and imagine yourself standing in your goal, or as Neville Goddard says, 'Standing there in the moment of the wish fulfilled.' Imagine that your Intention (what you want) is like the rudder of a ship. The focus of this is drawing you towards the result, steering you towards your destination.

Next, imagine how you will feel when you have achieved your goal; when you are right at that moment of achievement. Put all your attention inside yourself into this feeling. This feeling, this attention, is like the engine of a ship. The engine will help power the ship to its destination. Your desire of the goal, your wish, is like the high tide. It lifts you easily off and over the sand bar where you have been stuck.

Author of the book, *The Power of Awareness*, Neville says:

'Attention is forceful in proportion to narrowness. When you pay attention, it signifies that you have decided to focus your attention on one object or state rather than on another.'

When you create a habit of setting daily intentions, you are channelling your focus like a laser beam towards what you want. Send out what you want and it will be reflected back. In my experience, the more precisely and clearly you do this, the greater your likelihood of success.

AN EASY WAY TO REMEMBER INTENTIONS

I write my intentions on a card and carry them with me. On one side I write the intention and on the other side I write a question starting with how, such as *'How can I easily and effortlessly...* (Insert whatever it is I want to achieve.) Whenever I think about my intention I take the card out, read the intention, then the question and put it away again. Easy! It will help you stay on track.

For more help with writing intention cards, and other free tips, go to **http://www.mindsetforsuccess.com.au/getting-results-faster/**

POWER TIP

Developing your muscle of attention.

One technique to develop your attention muscle is the following exercise. Every night, before you drift off to sleep, dwell on the events of the day in reverse order. Focus your attention on the last thing you did, that is, getting into bed and then run your day backwards through each event until you reach the first event, getting out of bed.

Give it a go. See how far you get through this exercise before your mind wanders off on a tangent or you fall asleep. At first, it may only be a few seconds before your mind wanders. However, the more you practise this discipline, the more you work your muscle of attention.

Giving your brain a workout is also important in keeping yourself young and is a key to longevity. 'Use it or lose it' applies to the brain just as much as to your muscles when you are doing a physical workout.

YOUR IMAGINATION

HARNESSING THE AMAZING POWER OF YOUR IMAGINATION

'You can't do it unless you can imagine it.'
~ George Lucas

It has been estimated that we do about seventy per cent of our learning in the first six years of our life. We have an amazing capacity to absorb new things during this period and we have a very fertile imagination. When we get older, we tend to let our powers of imagination slip, letting it pull us over past memories or into the future, worrying about something that hasn't happened.

Our imagination is the key to all learning and solving problems. The Einsteins and Edisons of this world have all had excellent imaginations. Albert Einstein arrived at his scientific conclusions about time and space by mentally projecting himself out among the planets, where he would ride around on moonbeams! His ability to be childlike and 'dream big' helped him become a legend among intellectuals. The mind does not know what is real, imagined or pretend and as imagination uses the same neurological circuits as memory, when you vividly imagine what you want, you are giving instructions to your subconscious mind and recording it in your memory.

Now test how sharp your imagination is. Imagine eating a lemon right now. Can you feel and taste the tang in your mouth? Can you feel the sharpness of the juice? Does it make your mouth produce saliva? I have seen people scrunch their face up as they imagine the citrusy tang of the lemon in their mouth!

VISUALISATION HELPS ACHIEVE GOALS

Over the years, athletes have used visualisation to help them achieve their goals. I used to visualise myself running through the finish line at Forster, the Australian Ironman Championships. Night after night I imagined running through the finish line. I could see the time, I could hear the crowds cheering and I could feel the awesome feeling of finishing. Obviously, I took action (which is the bridge between our imagination and creating something) and committed to a training regime with a coach. I trained six days a week, consistently visualising the finish line. The more I did this, the more I built my belief. When race day came and I crossed the finish line, I knew this moment would happen because I had already seen it so many times in my mind.

TIME FOR ACTION:

Continue making a crystal clear picture about what you want and imagine it with full sensory detail daily. Feel the incredible feeling of having achieved what you want. Practise this technique, keeping your vision at the forefront of your mind, until it becomes part of your reality.

'All successful people, men and women are big dreamers. They imagine what their future could be, ideal in every respect and then they work every day toward their distant vision, that goal or purpose.'

~ Brian Tracy

CHOOSE TO BE HAPPIER!

WHAT REALLY MAKES YOU HAPPY?

'Happiness is not something ready made.
It comes from your own actions.'
~ Dalai Lama XIV

Perhaps the ultimate currency, the end toward which all other ends lead, is 'happiness'. Probably because of the flow-on effect on society as a whole, much research has been undertaken on the topic of Happiness. In 2012, the United Nations commissioned a report on World Happiness.

In Australia, we have an annual conference called 'Happiness and its causes', where questions up for discussion include:

> How should we live?

> How can happiness and wellbeing be increased?

> What creates satisfaction and meaning in life?

Some governments have commissioned reports on happiness. Bhutan measures their economy not by gross domestic product, but by Gross Domestic Happiness!

As our western way of life becomes busier and more people become depressed and unhappy, it appears that increasingly people are searching for more meaning in their life. They want to know how to simplify their lives and how to become happier.

Yet the study of happiness is certainly not unique to our society or post-modern age. Confucius walked from village to village to share his prescription for fulfilment; Plato institutionalised the study of the good life in his Academy and Aristotle opened the competing Lyceum to promote his own take on flourishing.

Tal Ben-Shahar, a lecturer in positive psychology at Harvard, has written an inspiring book called *Happier*. He defines happiness as, 'the overall experience of pleasure and meaning.' He goes onto say that, 'a happy person enjoys positive emotions while perceiving her life as purposeful.' It seems that combining activities that give us pleasure with attributing positive meanings to our actions and daily lives gives us joy. Happiness then becomes the experience of the journey rather than the destination.

HAPPINESS IS A CHOICE

Ultimately, happiness is a subjective feeling, or as Aristotle says, 'Happiness depends on ourselves'. So, at some level, we can choose to be happier whenever we want. If happiness is indeed an unlimited resource, we all have the innate capacity to tap into it and make it a lifelong pursuit to becoming happier.

Emotions cause motion and provide a motive that drives our actions. The word motive, source of motivation, comes from motivum, which means 'a moving cause'. In Latin, mover means 'to move' and the prefix 'e-' means 'away'. Emotions move us away from a desire-less state, providing us motivation to act! So, practise feeling good emotions and you have your own rule for taking action.

Past studies in the field of psychology have discussed a 'set point' of happiness. This set point is how you feel at a point in time. As the Dalai Lama says, 'choose to be optimistic, it feels better.'

HOW CAN YOU FEEL GOOD?

Simply by choosing good thoughts and thinking about things that make you happy! Specifically, you can reflect on past events that made you feel good. Or you can practise harnessing the power of your imagination to focus on what you want. Notice how that makes you feel.

Focus on how you will feel when you have created what you want.

When you feel good, it will be easier to continue taking the necessary action steps to achieve what you want.

Another way to tap into good feelings is to spend time focussing on what you are grateful for in your life. Bask in this feeling. This exercise will help you appreciate the positives in your life rather than take things for granted. According to research done by Robert Emmons and Michael McCullough, those who kept a journal, writing down daily at least five things for which they were grateful, enjoyed higher levels of emotional and physical wellbeing.

Consider the words people use when they are feeling good; words or phrases like, *'I am feeling on a high.'* Or, *'I am on top of the world.'* Or, *'I feel buzzing.'* When people feel down, they use words like, *'I am feeling down.'* Or, *'I am feeling flat today.'* As energy beings, we have different vibrational frequencies. The more you feel good energy, the more the hypothalamus in your brain can keep producing the good medicine, or higher vibrations which help you feel good. Consider the hypothalamus as a bit like your own pharmacy. When you feel good, it gives you a happy pill!

In the book *Happier*, Ben Tal Shahar mentions pleasurable experiences as a key to becoming happier. Taking time to do the things you love to do, like reading, exercising, being in nature, connecting with people and participating in other social or creative pursuits will make you feel good! This is backed up by Jiddu Krishnamurti, who wrote:

> *'You must understand the whole of life, not just one little part of it. That is why you must read, that is why you must look at the skies, that is why you must sing and dance, and write poems, and suffer, and understand for all that is life.'*

So, make sure you schedule in pursuits every week that are pleasurable to you.

The other component of being happier is the meaning you attribute to what you are doing or the meaning you put on your whole life. What do you do when something goes wrong? Do you think of the worst-case scenario? Will it be like a snowball, where this one event will create more of the same? Or do you choose to make light of it and move on? Do you begrudge your job or do you choose to make it meaningful to you? It's how you respond and react to life and events that contribute to your overall wellbeing and happiness.

When an event or experience doesn't go your way, start to cultivate a new habit by finding three or four different meanings to what just occurred. **Simply choose the meaning that gives you the best result.** When you do this, you will be able to make a better choice and determine what happens next. If you don't like your job, try to come up with a meaningful reason for doing it. At the very least, you will feel better about it!

There you have it. **It's inside you all the time**… the ability to feel good and be happier. So, keep practicing feeling good feelings and in time you will become happier. And when you are happier, you will be able to keep stepping forward towards the direction of your dreams.

COURAGE AND COMMITMENT

FLEXING YOUR MUSCLE OF COURAGE

'Our greatest weakness lies in giving up. The most certain way to succeed is always to try just one more time.'
~ Thomas A. Edison

Human nature is to resist change and to remain somewhere that is familiar and safe. This is commonly called 'the comfort zone'. Let me repeat what I said at the beginning.

Humans are creatures of habit and are hardwired to be kept safe.

Unless you consistently step out of your comfort zone, you will not achieve the level of success or growth you desire. You will remain in your comfort zone or fall back into it. This is the main reason why people don't change, fall back into old ways or let their best plans dissolve. It takes effort and courage, both of which go against our safety programs! This is why taking small steps and creating rituals are keys in carving habits that serve your future successes.

DO YOU SIMPLY NEED WILLPOWER?

I often hear people say they lack willpower, justifying why they can't change. However, willpower and courage are part of the same muscle. When you exercise your muscle of courage, you are building your willpower. When your willpower builds, it's easier to keep going and to work your muscle of courage. When you exercise your muscle of courage, you build your belief. They all work together.

In an interview with the swim coach Stephan Widmer, Stephan talked about the importance of setting his athletes small challenges daily and weekly. Over time, the fruition of these small challenges built a solid foundation of self-belief, self-esteem and personal power (ingredients to success!) He helped Libby Trickett and Leisel Jones win Olympic gold medals in swimming. Read the full interview here: **http://www.mindsetforsuccess.com.au/olympic-swim-coach-shares-success-insights/**

If they can win gold medals in their chosen sport, imagine what you can achieve in your life when you set yourself small challenges every day. They don't have to be physical challenges either, even though these are definitely a proven way to build personal belief. It could simply be to write ten pages per day of your book.

Growth happens when you extend yourself and 'push' yourself out of your comfort zone. Of course it's difficult at first due to fear and doubt. But most of the time, what we fear is just a construct of the mind and it's never as scary as we once thought!

Ralph Waldo Emerson said, 'The mind, once stretched by a new idea, never returns to its original dimensions.' A diamond, once formed, can never return to being coal either. So stretch yourself and transform your life!

In the words of Apollinaire:

'Come to the edge. We can't we're afraid. Come to the edge. We can't we'll fall. Come to the edge. And they came to the edge and he pushed them. And they flew.'

COMMIT TO YOUR OWN SUCCESS

To ensure you create new healthy habits and lock them in, you must be committed to your own success. You must choose what you want to do or become in accordance with your own goals, values and passions.

You must also find meaning and pleasure in what you do. An accountant who finds meaning and pleasure in her work, who is in it for the right reasons, leads a more fulfilling life than a monk or a priest who is in his field for the wrong reasons.

To stay committed to the journey, you need to create daily rituals and practise mental disciplines. With consistent steps and continued action, you will create new neural connections, which then become your habits.

Finally, remember to celebrate your successes! Your brain loves rewards. When you celebrate your successes, however big or small, your brain will reward you with a shot of dopamine, the 'happy' hormone. As I mentioned earlier, success is the fuel for more success.

When you are happy with who you are and you are living a pleasurable and meaningful life, you will feel more fulfilled. When you learn to let go of negative meanings, judgments and self-criticism, you will become more at peace. You will be living in the moment and being more present.

It is the sum total of the choices you make every moment of your life that will determine your future successes and results.

'In the space between yes and no, there's a lifetime. It's the difference between the path you walk and the one you leave behind; it's the gap between who you thought you could be and who you really are; it's the legroom for the lies you'll tell yourself in the future.'

~ Jodi Picoult, Change of Heart

THE HABIT CHANGER PLAN

A STEP-BY-STEP GUIDE
TO GETTING STARTED

'Success seems to be connected with action.
Successful people keep moving. They make
mistakes, but they don't quit.'

~ Conrad Hilton

Here is a step-by-step summary of how to get started and use the information in this book in a sequential order.

Select one area of your life that needs some attention. Get clear as to what isn't working and what you want by changing.

Write a clear goal and break it down into action steps or tasks. Schedule the tasks into your diary. Create rituals that will help you move forward.

Monitor your self-talk and change it if it isn't positive. This needs to be mastered until it is natural to only talk positively about what you want.

Set daily intentions that will help you keep on track and inspired to keep moving in the direction of your dreams and goals.

Write out a mantra or positive statement that will help you become the person you want to be to achieve what you want. For example it might be: 'I am confident and calmer every day.' Or, 'Every day it is becoming easier to select healthy food choices.'

Find someone to hold you accountable – a friend, family member or an expert in the field of change and transformation.

When you have made 3 or 4 habits, practise the art of visualising what you want.

Write down your successes daily and celebrate!

Practise giving three meanings to your experiences and choose the one that gives you the best results and supports you in the best manner. Watch your world change in a positive way.

Review your week and check your progress. Remember to reward yourself along the way.

Keep going and pick another area of your life to focus on.

In the words of Einstein:

'I must be willing to give up what I am in order to become what I will be.'

YOUR HABIT CHANGER PLAN

If you'd like a personalised plan for creating healthier habits, either through personal or online coaching programs, please visit my website **http://www.mindsetforsuccess.com.au or email info@mindsetforsuccess.com.au**.

BONUS TOOLS

TRANSFORMING AND DISSOLVING
A PROBLEM

'Challenges are part of life.
Overcoming them is dependant on what you
interpret them to mean.'
~ Mandy Napier

When you make changes to your old patterns, habits and ways of being, be aware that obstacles and rocks will appear. This is life. We are cyclical, like the seasons and the oceans. If you surf, sometimes the waves are perfect, sometimes there are no waves and sometimes they are just too big for your level of experience! **So it just is.** Problems in life appear and disappear. It's what we do with the problem, how we choose to deal with it that counts.

Use this process to chip away at your problems… your roadblocks to success. You can use it to help dissolve your overwhelming feeling, procrastination or stress. You can use it to release a negative emotion or anytime you can't find a solution to a problem you are facing.

HOW TO DO THE PROCESS

Practise changing your focus. **Pick a spot on a wall at eye level.** Put all of your attention and awareness onto the spot and 'stare' at it! You are now in what we call 'foveal vision'.

As you remain focussed on this spot, **move your attention outwards, towards the periphery.** Notice how you can see out to the side and allow your vision to expand, as if you can almost see behind you. Keep resting your eyes on the spot as you do this. You are now in what we call 'Expanded awareness'.

Now just **relax your eyes and look away**. Easy!

Associate with a problem you have. Imagine the entire problem is contained in the spot on the wall. While focussing totally on the spot, 'dump' the entire problem onto the spot, verbally, (or to yourself if there are people around). Talk the entire problem out and then ask the following questions: 'What is the problem?' 'How is it a problem for me right now in my life?' 'What has it been preventing me from doing, being or having?' 'How will it continue to be a problem if I hold onto it?' Dump all aspects of the problem out onto the spot.

Once you have 'dumped' the problem, **shift all of your attention to the periphery,** while still resting your eyes on the spot. Sit quietly for a moment and ask yourself, 'What positive learnings for myself can I take right now, that will allow me to easily and effortlessly release the problem?'

Observe what happens next. Trust the process. Something will pop up. It might be a word, a phrase, a feeling or picture. It might be something that seems so simple you tend to overlook it. Whatever it is for you, trust that it will be perfect.

From what you observe, select the one thing that if you chose to believe it, would get the biggest results in your life. Then take action on one thing immediately. This will change your focus and empower you to be able to act in a more positive manner!

VISUALISATION FOR CREATING CHANGE

'Imagination get you from A to B.
Imagination will take you everywhere.'
~ Einstein

WHAT DO YOU WANT?

> An ideal relationship?

> To get that overseas job or promotion?

> To become optimally healthy or reach your ideal weight?

Whatever it is, visualisation can help you. The example below outlines how to visualise for weight loss, because I am often working with clients who struggle to lose weight and maintain their ideal weight.

Imagine you are communicating with someone who doesn't speak your language.

How would you communicate with them? One effective way is to use the universal language of pictures. If you needed to find a toilet, you could draw a picture of one and most people would know what you were looking for! In the same manner, you can use visualisation to communicate with your own brain. When you use your imagination to create a visual image of a thinner person, or you at your ideal weight, you are beginning to create a new inner program.

With repetition, this picture becomes etched into your subconscious mind, which gives it something to focus on. When you add other necessary action steps, such as exercising, eating healthily, clearing out old beliefs, clearing unwanted emotions, changing strategies and behaviours about food and eating, then you are well on your way to success. Make sure your action plan includes regular exercise and a good eating regime! Plenty of fresh fruit and vegetables, organic if possible. **Eliminate as many processed foods as possible**. These all contain chemicals that inhibit your body's ability to lose weight and clog up your liver, preventing it from working on what it is supposed to do, breaking down fats in your body.

The best time to practise visualising is first thing in the morning or last thing at night. At this time, you are generally relaxing and resting and your internal chatter is quieter. Your ability to focus and create a visual image will be stronger which means so will the message you send to your subconscious mind.

Imagine looking at a reflection in a still pond. **In the stillness you will see a mirror image in the pond**. If there is wind, there will be ripples, which will distort the image. It will not be so perfect.

Your subconscious mind is the same. When it is quiet it is like a pond with no ripples. It can clearly see the image you are trying to create. When your mind is busy with thoughts there will be too many thought waves distorting the image and you won't be able to see it clearly.

HOW DO WE VISUALISE?

Whilst resting in bed, visualise yourself as clearly as you can looking exactly as you would like to look. Make the picture as real as possible by adding in a specific place, time or event.

> Where will you be?

> What will you be wearing?

> Who will be there with you?

> What you will be saying to yourself?

> What will you be feeling when you are in this moment?

Hear the sounds as if you are right there. Smell the air, feel the sun or wind on your body as if you were right there. Taste the spray of the ocean if you are near it, or feel the salt on your skin. Create a clear picture of what is going on. If you are celebrating, how you will be celebrating? If you are opening up a bottle of champagne, hear the cork pop, see the champagne flow into the glasses, taste the bubbles in your mouth and savour the magic of the moment.

Make sure that wherever you are, be there in that moment, with all your senses and notice how it feels absolutely real. Perhaps you are congratulating yourself, saying, 'This is who I am, this is me. I love my body.' Whatever you say, feel it to be true with absolute certainty. Decide to do this, commit, take action and practise. Practise some more and then some more.

Deepak Chopra, in his book *The Seven Spiritual Laws of Success,* talks about the 'Laws of Pure Potentiality' and 'The Law of Intention and Desire'. He believes we can manifest anything in our lives by taking intention or desire into the 'field of pure potentiality'.

The intention is our image of how we want to look. When you are in the relaxed state (last thing at night or first thing in the morning) you are entering the **'field of pure potentiality'**.

You are visualising what you want and actively creating the 'body of your dreams'.

Practising the art of visualisation helps you create what you want in your external world. You can use visualisation for improved performance, creating confidence in exams, at an interview, or for becoming a more efficient worker. I teach athletes how to visualise their perfect race and businessmen and women how to visualise themselves being confident at public speaking. And we all know that practice isn't something you do once you are good. It's something you do that helps make you good!

So, it is up to you. Will you act upon the information in this book? Will you remember the tools and use them to make the changes you desire in your life? Will you persist in understanding yourself and how you function and invest in your future self? Or, will you succumb to your current conditioning, remaining a creature of habit and settle for less?

It is my wish that you act and open yourself up to your limitless potential.

It's your life. It's your choice. What will you choose?

ABOUT THE AUTHOR

Mandy Napier, dubbed the 'Mindset Alchemist,' helps people harness the power of their minds, change their current results and live happier, healthier lives. She has assisted more than 1,000 clients to clear their blocks, get out of their own way and literally re-wire themselves for success.

Having represented Australia four times in ultra-distance Ironman competitions, Mandy Napier understands what it takes to achieve goals, dreams and personal fulfilment. Early on, Mandy's dream to ride horses inspired her to find many productive ways to afford a horse and to compete at a county level.

This entrepreneurial streak also helped fund her travels from London to Asia and on to Australia after graduating University. She easily transitioned into management and leadership roles and immersed herself in personal development and human behaviour, including becoming a Master Practitioner and Trainer of Neuro-Linguistic Programming and Hypnosis.

Mandy has used these experiences in life and her commitment to excellence to create her own system of coaching, the C.L.E.A.R™ Coaching Model. Testament to its effectiveness is that she has worked with all kinds of people nationally and internationally, from individuals in large organisations such as BHP Billiton, to entrepreneurs, managers, small business owners, teams and life coaches. Clients often state how they have gone from being 'stuck' or 'stale' in life to feeling more capable, lighter and freer, while others have been amazed at the life changing transformations they have experienced as they tap into their limitless potential.

As a Mindset Specialist and Performance Coach, Mandy loves to share her knowledge and expertise in human behaviour and how to create change through writing eBooks, magazine articles, producing hypnosis audio programs and keynote speaking. Her tenacious spirit, determination to help others succeed, along with her proprietary mindset coaching system, means Mandy Napier is an authentic leader in her field.

Mandy takes time out in her busy schedule to practice Ashtanga yoga and enjoys running and swimming in the ocean. She loves travelling with her husband William, who is often found in their garden, growing and cultivating fresh produce, before creating delicious healthy meals.

Mandy's most popular speaking topics are:

> **Setting Yourself Up With a Mindset for Success - Re-wiring your brain for optimal business performance**

> The Winning (W)edge

> The Art of Being HAPPIER!

> Transforming Stress Into Success

YOU CAN CONNECT WITH MANDY NAPIER BY:

Phone:	+61 7 408 666 176
Email:	info@mindsetforsuccess.com.au
Post:	Mindset for Success
	P.O. Box 132, Golden Beach
	QLD 4551, Australia
Facebook:	www.facebook.com/mindsetforsuccess11
Linked In:	www.linkedin.com/in/mandynapier

BONUS OFFER:

If you would like to get started on your journey of transformation today, contact Mandy to book in for your Success Strategy Session. The special price for readers of this book is only $95. (Normally $210). There are four available every month and can be conducted via Skype worldwide. Please mention this offer when booking. If self-paced online coaching sounds appealing, **visit www.mindsetforsuccess.com.au/90-day-online-coaching/**

MORE RESOURCES

> **Visit www.mindsetforsuccess.com. au** to access free E book 'Your Hidden Mind' and receive monthly mindset tips.

> **To purchase books, hypnosis audios and for information on workshops,** visit www.mindsetforsuccess.com.au and click on the products tab.

> **For information regarding Mandy Napier's Mindset for Success® Coaching** and how it can help you create the life you desire, please email **info@mindsetforsuccess.com.au**

> **Personalised programs, online coaching and group coaching options are available.**

Mandy Napier's
MINDSET
for Success®
EMPOWERMENT. ACTION. RESULTS.

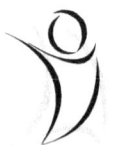

*'If you are not consciously directing your life,
you will lose your footing and circumstances
will decide for you.'*

~ Michael Bernard Beckwith